DAILY STRETCHES ROUTINE

ELIZABETH JONAH

Table of Contents

Chapter 1: Introduction to Daily Stretching

A daily stretches routine is a technique that includes practicing a set of stretching exercises frequently, often on a daily basis. The fundamental objective of daily stretches is to increase flexibility, enhance muscle and joint mobility, and promote general physical well-being. Here's what daily stretches are all about:

1. Flexibility: Daily stretches are aimed to develop your flexibility, which refers to the range of motion in your joints and muscles. Improved flexibility may lead to improved posture, lower chance of injury, and greater sports performance.

2. Muscle Health: Stretching helps relax and lengthen muscles. It may ease muscular tension, reduce pain, and avoid muscle imbalances, which might arise due to everyday activity or repeated motions.

3. Joint Mobility: Stretching exercises target the joints as well. Regular stretching may promote joint mobility, making it simpler to accomplish everyday chores and maintain a broad range of motion as you age.

4. Stress Reduction: Stretching may have a relaxing impact on the body and mind. It may help decrease

tension, induce relaxation, and increase mental clarity, making it a significant aspect of stress management.

5. Posture Improvement: Daily stretches help repair bad posture by targeting muscles that can be tight or weak. This may lead to improved alignment and less strain on the spine and supporting muscles.

6. Injury Prevention: A flexible and well-conditioned body is less prone to injuries. Daily stretches may help avoid common ailments including strains, sprains, and muscle pulls.

7. Enhanced Performance: For athletes and fitness aficionados, frequent stretching may boost athletic performance by enhancing muscle function, increasing agility, and minimizing the risk of overuse injuries.

8. Rehabilitation: Stretching may be a crucial component of injury rehabilitation. It may assist in the rehabilitation process by boosting healing, restoring range of motion, and reducing muscular atrophy during times of immobility.

9. Overall Well-Being: Incorporating regular stretches into your routine may lead to an enhanced overall feeling of well-being. It may enhance energy levels, relieve stress, and improve circulation.

10. Long-Term Health: Maintaining flexibility and joint mobility via regular stretching may have long-term

health advantages, such as lowering the risk of age-related disorders like osteoarthritis.

In short, a daily stretching practice is about taking proactive actions to preserve and increase your physical health and well-being. It's a simple but powerful practice that can be adapted to your unique needs and objectives, whether you're wanting to decrease stiffness, develop flexibility, heal from an accident, or simply feel better in your everyday life.

- The Importance of Daily Stretching

The value of regular stretching cannot be emphasized, as it delivers several physical and mental advantages that contribute to overall health and well-being. Here are some significant reasons showing the relevance of including regular stretching into your routine:

1. Improved Flexibility: Stretching exercises assist to enhance the flexibility of muscles and joints. This greater flexibility boosts your range of motion, making it simpler to conduct everyday tasks and minimizing the chance of muscle strains and joint problems.

2. Enhanced Posture: Daily stretching helps address muscular imbalances and ease stress in regions prone to poor posture, such as the neck, shoulders, and lower back. This, in turn, may lead to improved alignment and reduced tension on the spine.

3. Reduced muscular Tension: Stretching relaxes and lengthens muscles, decreasing muscular tension and stiffness. This may be especially good for people who spend long hours sitting at a desk or engaged in repetitive tasks.

4. Stress Reduction: Stretching may have a relaxing impact on the body and mind. It promotes relaxation, decreases stress hormones, and may increase mental clarity and attention. Incorporating stretching into your daily routine may help manage stress and improve a feeling of well-being.

5. Injury Prevention: Regular stretching may strengthen the suppleness of muscles and tendons, minimizing the risk of injury during physical activity. It also helps to maintain muscular balance, minimizing overuse injuries and strains.

6. Improved Circulation: Stretching improves blood flow to the muscles, which may help in the supply of nutrients and oxygen. This increased circulation leads to muscle rehabilitation and general cardiovascular health.

7. Pain Management: For persons with chronic pain disorders, such as back pain or arthritis, mild stretching may give relief by improving joint mobility and lowering muscle tightness.

8. Better Athletic Performance: Athletes typically include stretching into their everyday routines to boost performance. Stretching increases muscular function, agility, and coordination, which may lead to greater athletic outcomes and decreased risk of sports-related injuries.

9. Joint Health: Stretching exercises target the joints as well, helping to preserve joint mobility and lower the risk of disorders like osteoarthritis. It may help reduce joint stiffness, which is typical as individuals age.

10. Long-Term Health: Consistent daily stretching may help to long-term health and energy. It may assist preserve physical function as you age, minimizing the risk of mobility difficulties and falls in older persons.

11. Relaxation and Mindfulness: Stretching may be a mindful activity, helping you to connect with your body and become more aware of physical sensations. This mindfulness element may induce relaxation and a feeling of well-being.

In conclusion, regular stretching is a simple but effective activity that gives a broad variety of physical and mental advantages. Whether you're wanting to develop flexibility, decrease stress, avoid injuries, or boost your general quality of life, including regular stretching into your routine may be a helpful and enjoyable habit.

- Benefits of Incorporating Stretching into Your Routine

Incorporating stretching into your daily routine provides a range of advantages that may enhance your physical and emotional well-being. Here are some of the primary benefits of making stretching a regular part of your everyday activities:

1. Greater Flexibility: Stretching exercises assist to enhance the length and suppleness of your muscles, leading to greater flexibility. This expanded range of motion makes it simpler to do routine chores and participate in physical activities without pain or limits.

2. Reduced muscular Tension: Stretching may relax tight muscles and reduce muscular tension. This is especially advantageous if you have a sedentary work or indulge in activities that contribute to muscular tightness.

3. Enhanced Range of Motion: Regular stretching may boost joint mobility and extend your range of motion. This is particularly crucial for maintaining optimum

function in your joints, which may avoid joint-related disorders as you age.

4. Better Posture: Stretching helps address muscular imbalances and release stress in regions prone to bad posture, such as the neck, shoulders, and lower back. This may lead to better alignment and less strain on the spine.

5. Injury Prevention: Stretching before physical activity helps warm up your muscles and prepare them for effort, minimizing the chance of muscle strains and ligament sprains. It also Improves greater muscular balance, lowering the incidence of overuse problems.

6. Stress Reduction: Stretching may have a relaxing impact on the neurological system. It induces relaxation, decreases stress hormones, and may increase mental clarity and attention, making it a useful stress management strategy.

7. Enhanced Circulation: Stretching improves blood flow to the muscles, which may help in the supply of nutrients and oxygen. This increased circulation leads to muscle rehabilitation and general cardiovascular health.

8. Pain Relief: For persons with chronic pain disorders, such as back pain or arthritis, stretching may give relief by improving joint mobility and lowering muscle tightness.

9. Better Athletic Performance: Athletes typically include stretching into their regimens to boost performance. Stretching increases muscular function, agility, and coordination, which may lead to greater athletic outcomes and decreased risk of sports-related injuries.

10. Joint Health: Stretching activities target the joints as well, helping to preserve joint mobility and lower the risk of disorders like osteoarthritis. It may help reduce joint stiffness, which is typical as individuals age.

11. Mindfulness and Relaxation: Stretching may be a thoughtful exercise, helping you to connect with your body and become more aware of physical sensations. This mindfulness element may induce relaxation and a feeling of well-being.

12. Long-Term Health: Consistent stretching may help to long-term health and energy. It may assist preserve physical function as you age, minimizing the risk of mobility difficulties and falls in older persons.

Incorporating stretching into your regular routine doesn't need a big-time investment and can be done practically anyplace. Whether you're wanting to better your athletic performance, decrease stress, avoid injuries, or just improve your general quality of life, the advantages of regular stretching are well worth the effort.

Common Misconceptions about Stretching

Stretching is a widespread activity in fitness and health regimens, but there are various misunderstandings and myths surrounding it. Understanding these myths is vital for safe and successful stretching. Here are some typical misunderstandings regarding stretching:

1. Stretching Should Always Be Done Before Exercise: One of the most popular fallacies is that you should always stretch before exercise. While it's vital to warm up before severe activity, static stretching (holding a stretch for a lengthy time) before exercise may actually diminish muscle strength and function. It's advisable to undertake dynamic warm-up activities before a workout and preserve static stretching for later or during cooldown.

2. Stretching Prevents Muscle Soreness: Stretching may not prevent delayed onset muscle soreness (DOMS) after intensive activity. While it may aid with immediate relaxation of muscular tension, it may not considerably diminish soreness that develops 24-48 hours following activity. Other healing techniques, including rest, hydration, and good diet, have a more substantial role in controlling DOMS.

3. The More You Stretch, the Better: Overstretching or excessive stretching may lead to damage. Pushing oneself too far in a stretch may tear muscles and ligaments. It's crucial to stretch within your limitations and move gradually to prevent harm.

4. Stretching Will Make You More Flexible Overnight: Gaining flexibility requires time and persistence. Stretching occasionally or seldom won't result in instant increases in flexibility. It needs frequent practice over a prolonged time to notice major increases in flexibility.

5. Stretching Should Be unpleasant: Stretching should never be unpleasant. A minor discomfort or stretching feeling is acceptable, but if you experience severe or strong pain, you should stop immediately. Stretching should be a calm and regulated action.

6. Stretching may Undo Poor Posture: While stretching may assist rectify muscular imbalances associated with poor posture, it may not be adequate on its own. Addressing posture typically includes strengthening workouts in addition to stretching.

7. Stretching Before Bed Improves Sleep: While stretching may help calm the body and mind, it's not a guarantee of better sleep. Other variables, such as sleep hygiene routines, stress management, and a suitable sleep environment, have a more substantial impact in increasing sleep quality.

8. Stretching Prevents Injuries Completely: While frequent stretching may lessen the risk of certain injuries, it doesn't ensure total injury avoidance. Injury prevention also relies on elements including good technique, fitness, and rest.

9. Only Muscles Need Stretching: Stretching may also help connective tissues, such as tendons and fascia, which can enhance joint mobility and general flexibility. It's not only about stretching muscles.

10. One Type of Stretching Fits All: There are numerous forms of stretching, including static, dynamic, ballistic, and PNF (proprioceptive neuromuscular facilitation) stretching. The sort of stretching you should perform depends on your objectives and the circumstances (e.g., pre-workout warm-up vs. post-workout cooldown).

Understanding these misunderstandings might help you approach stretching more successfully and safely. It's vital to personalize your stretching practice to your unique requirements, listen to your body, and seek help from fitness experts or physical therapists if you have specific objectives or problems.

Chapter 2: Getting Started with Daily Stretches

- Setting Your Stretching Goals

Setting specific and attainable stretching objectives is vital to make the most of your stretching program and measure your progress over time. Whether you're aiming to increase flexibility, decrease muscular tension, or target particular areas of pain, here's a step-by-step guide on how to develop successful stretching goals:

1. Identify Your Motivation: - Start by understanding why you want to add stretching into your routine. Is it to improve sports performance, ease muscular stiffness, reduce stress, boost posture, or treat a particular ailment like lower back pain? Knowing your motivation will help you develop meaningful objectives.

2. Make Your Goals Specific: - Clearly outline your stretching goals. Instead of a general objective like "I want to be more flexible," clarify what that means for you. For example, "I want to touch my toes without discomfort" or "I want to increase my shoulder mobility to perform overhead exercises with ease."

3. Set Measurable Goals: - Make your objectives quantifiable so you can measure your progress. Use measurable measures or benchmarks, such as attaining a given degree of flexibility in inches, holding a stretch for a specified length, or accomplishing a particular range of motion in a joint.

4. Establish a Timeline: - Determine a suitable timeline during which you want to attain your stretching objectives. Having a deadline might help you remain motivated and focused. Be realistic about the time it may take to see meaningful improvement, since flexibility increases might vary from person to person.

5. Break Goals into Smaller Steps: - Large stretching goals might be scary. Break things down into tiny, doable stages or milestones. This makes the process more attainable and helps you to appreciate your success along the way.

6. Prioritize and Sequence: - If you have many stretching objectives, rank them based on significance and relevance. Consider arranging your objectives to work on one at a time or in a logical manner that avoids interference between goals.

7. Consider Your existing Ability: - Assess your existing degree of flexibility and mobility in the areas connected to your objectives. This baseline measurement will let you monitor development correctly.

8. **Select right Stretching methods**: - Choose the right stretching methods that match with your aims. For example, if you intend to develop static flexibility, concentrate on static stretching. If you wish to promote joint mobility, try dynamic stretches or yoga-based stretches.

9. Create a Structured Plan: - Develop an organized stretching plan that describes the particular stretches, sets, repetitions, and frequency necessary to reach your objectives. A well-organized strategy guarantees you're continually working toward your goals.

10. Track and Adjust: - Keep a stretching notebook or use a tracking app to document your improvement. Regularly analyze if you're making advances toward your objectives. If required, adapt your strategy depending on your findings and any input from your body.

11. Seek Professional instruction: - If you have special objectives relating to injury rehabilitation, sports performance, or complicated flexibility difficulties, consider visiting a physical therapist, athletic trainer, or skilled fitness professional for individualized instruction and help.

Remember that perseverance and patience are crucial while working towards stretching objectives. As you make progress, evaluate and update your objectives to continue pushing yourself and preserving your flexibility improvements.

- Creating a Consistent Routine

Creating a regular stretching regimen is vital for attaining your flexibility and mobility objectives. A consistent practice ensures that you make stretching a habit and get its advantages over time. Here's a step-by-step tutorial on how to begin and maintain a regular stretching routine:

1. Define Your Goals: - As discussed previously, define your stretching objectives. Knowing what you want to accomplish helps offer motivation and direction for your workout.

2. Select a Convenient Time: - Choose a time of day that works best for you and your schedule. Some individuals like stretching in the morning to launch their day, while others find it useful before or after exercises, or even before night for relaxation. Consistency is crucial, so select a time that you can commit to consistently.

3. Start Small: - If you're new to stretching or re-establishing a habit, start with a modest time. Aim for

only a few minutes of stretching each day, gradually increasing the duration as your flexibility and comfort improve.

4. Create a Dedicated Space: - Designate a pleasant and clutter-free space where you may stretch. Having a specific place might help you get into the regular mentality.

5. Set Reminders: - Use reminders, alarms, or calendar alerts to urge you to stretch at your selected time. Consistency typically takes subtle nudges, particularly when you're creating a new habit.

6. Plan Your Stretches: - Develop an organized stretching routine that includes a range of stretches targeting various muscle groups or areas of concentration. Plan your program in advance so you know what stretches to execute each day.

7. Mix It Up: - To minimize boredom and plateaus, modify your stretches often. Incorporate diverse forms of stretching, such as static, dynamic, or yoga-based stretches, into your practice. This keeps your workout fresh and pushes your body in new ways.

8. Listen to Your Body: - Pay attention to how your body reacts to stretching. Stretch to the point of moderate discomfort but avoid pushing yourself into agony. It's crucial to practice safe and efficient stretching practices to prevent injury.

9. Consistency Over Intensity: - Consistency is more crucial than intensity. It's best to perform shorter, less difficult stretches routinely than occasional intensive bouts. Gradual development is safer and more sustainable.

10. monitor Your Progress: - Keep a stretching notebook or use a mobile app to record your daily stretching sessions and monitor your progress toward your objectives. This might be inspiring and help you remain on track.

11. Reward Yourself: - Celebrate your successes and milestones. Reward yourself for sticking to your regimen or accomplishing certain flexibility objectives. Positive reinforcement may help retain your motivation.

12. Accountability Partner: - Consider stretching with a buddy or partner. Having someone to stretch with might make it more pleasurable and help you remain responsible.

13. Adapt to Life Changes: - Life may be unexpected. If you miss a stretching practice due to unexpected circumstances, don't be disheartened. Simply continue your routine the following day. Consistency doesn't demand perfection.

14. Stay Informed: - Stay current on stretching methods, best practices, and any alterations to your program that may be required to reach your objectives.

15. Evaluate and alter: - Periodically examine your stretching program and alter it as appropriate. As your flexibility and objectives change, your routine may need to adjust as well.

Remember that consistency is the key to success with stretching. Over time, you'll enjoy the advantages of better flexibility, less muscular tension, and enhanced general well-being.

- Finding the Right Time and Place

Finding the correct time and location for your stretching regimen is vital for building a regular and successful practice. Here are some guidelines to help you choose the ideal time and place for your stretching sessions:

1. Consider Your routine: - Evaluate your daily routine to discover moments when you have unbroken periods accessible for stretching. Choose a time that is reasonable and possible for you. It might be in the morning, at a lunch break, after work, or before night.

2. Align with Your Natural Rhythms: - Pay attention to your body's natural rhythms. Some individuals feel that stretching in the morning helps wake them up and invigorate them for the day, while others prefer nighttime stretching to unwind and relax before sleep.

3. Coordinate with Workouts: - If you have a regular workout program, try integrating stretching either as part of your warm-up or cooldown. Stretching after exercises may be especially effective for increasing flexibility and lowering muscular tension.

4. Create a Dedicated Space: - Choose a spot where you can comfortably execute your stretching regimen. Ideally, this environment should be peaceful, well-ventilated, and free from interruptions. Having a distinct location for stretching might help you psychologically prepare for your practice.

5. Adapt to Your Surroundings: - If you have limited room, alter your stretching exercise appropriately. You may practice sitting stretches or concentrate on stretches that need minimum space. The goal is to make the most of the surroundings you have.

6. Use Props and Equipment: - Depending on your selected stretches, you may require props like yoga mats, foam rollers, or resistance bands. Ensure that you have easy access to the appropriate equipment in your selected location.

7. Account for Privacy: - If privacy is essential to you, pick a spot where you can stretch without feeling self-conscious or noticed. This may be especially significant for some yoga postures or stretches that need more open body positions.

8. Minimize Distractions: - Find an area that minimizes distractions. Turn off your phone or set it on quiet mode during your stretching sessions to really immerse yourself in the activity.

9. Experiment and Adjust: - It may take some trial to discover the exact time and location that works best for you. Be open to modifying your routine if you learn that your first option doesn't correspond with your requirements or preferences.

10. Be Consistent: - Once you've chosen the perfect time and location, keep to your schedule regularly. Consistency is crucial to obtaining the advantages of stretching.

11. try Outdoor Options: - If you like the outdoors, try stretching in a park or garden. Outdoor places may give a pleasant change of view and provide natural factors like fresh air and sunshine.

Ultimately, the proper time and location for your stretching routine should correspond with your personal preferences, daily schedule, and the objectives you've established for your stretching practice. By establishing a proper location and adding stretching into your daily routine, you may make it a lasting and healthy habit.

- Essential Equipment and Attire

When it comes to everyday stretching activities, having the correct equipment and apparel may boost your comfort and efficacy throughout your practice. Here's a list of needed equipment and clothes for an effective stretching routine:

1. Comfortable clothes: - Wear comfortable, breathable clothes that allows for a complete range of motion. Opt for moisture-wicking textiles that assist keep you dry if you sweat throughout your stretching workouts.

2. Athletic Shoes or Barefoot: - Depending on your stretching practice, you may either conduct stretches barefoot or wear sports shoes with sufficient arch support. Yoga and mat-based stretches are frequently done barefoot, but certain dynamic stretches may necessitate shoes.

3. Yoga Mat: - A yoga mat offers a pleasant and non-slip surface for different stretching activities. It's particularly handy for floor-based stretches and yoga positions.

Look for a mat that meets your demands in terms of thickness and texture.

4. Towel or Yoga Blanket: - A small towel or yoga blanket may be helpful for giving padding and support during stretches, particularly if you're practicing sitting or lying stretches.

5. Stretching Strap or Resistance Band: - A stretching strap or resistance band may aid in reaching deeper stretches and increasing flexibility. These gadgets are especially beneficial for leg and hamstring stretches.

6. Foam Roller: - A foam roller is good for self-myofascial release (self-massage) and may help reduce muscular tension and increase flexibility. It's typically utilized as part of a pre-stretching warm-up or post-stretching cooldown.

7. Yoga Blocks: - Yoga blocks are beneficial for adjusting yoga positions and giving support during stretches. They may help you maintain appropriate alignment and progressively build toward more demanding stretches.

8. Comfortable Surface: - If you're stretching on a hard surface, you may wish to use a cushion or workout mat to prevent your knees and joints from pain.

9. Water Bottle: - Staying hydrated is vital, especially during stretching activities. Have a water bottle available

to keep yourself hydrated, particularly if you're completing a lengthy workout.

10. Timer or Stopwatch: - A timer or stopwatch may help you monitor the length of your stretches, ensuring you hold each stretch for the optimum period of time. Many cell phones have built-in timers that you may utilize.

11. Music or Relaxation Aids: - Consider playing soothing music or utilizing relaxation aids like peaceful smells or guided meditation recordings if you find it helps you relax while stretching.

12. Mirror: - Having a full-length mirror may be excellent for checking your form and alignment during stretches, particularly if you're new to stretching or practicing yoga postures.

13. Resistance Bands with Handles: - For strength and flexibility training, resistance bands with handles may provide diversity to your stretching practice, enabling you to target various muscle areas.

14. Stability Ball: - A stability ball may be utilized for many stretches, particularly those that entail balance and core activation.

Remember that the particular equipment you require may vary depending on your stretching objectives and the sort of stretches you're completing. Having the correct clothes and equipment may make your stretching regimen more pleasurable and productive while lowering the chance of injury.

Chapter 3: Key Stretches for Daily Routine

- Neck and Shoulder Stretches

Stretching the neck and shoulders is vital for alleviating tension, increasing flexibility, and minimizing pain caused by bad posture or stress. Here are some helpful neck and shoulder exercises to integrate into your everyday routine:

1. Neck Tilt Stretch:
- Sit or stand with your back straight.
- Slowly tilt your head to one side, bringing your ear nearer your shoulder.
- Hold the stretch for 15-30 seconds.
- Repeat on the opposite side.
- Perform 2-3 repetitions on each side.

2. Neck Rotation Stretch:

- Sit or stand with your back straight.
- Slowly shift your head to one side, gazing over your shoulder.
- Hold the stretch for 15-30 seconds.
- Repeat on the opposite side.
- Perform 2-3 repetitions on each side.

3. Neck Flexor Stretch:
- Sit or stand with your back straight.
- Gently tilt your head forward, bringing your chin closer to your chest.
- Hold the stretch for 15-30 seconds.
- You may intensify the stretch by exerting gentle pressure with your palm on the back of your head.
- Release and return to the starting position.
- Perform 2-3 repetitions.

4. Neck Extensor Stretch:
- Sit or stand with your back straight.
- Gently tilt your head backward, facing upward.
- Hold the stretch for 15-30 seconds.
- You may support your head with your hand for a deeper stretch.
- Release and return to the starting position.
- Perform 2-3 repetitions.

5. Shoulder Roll:
- Sit or stand with your back straight.
- Roll your shoulders forward in a circular manner.
- Complete 10-15 forward rolls.

- Reverse the action and roll your shoulders backward for 10-15 repetitions.

6. Neck and Shoulder Stretch Combo:
- Sit or stand with your back straight.
- Place your right hand behind your back, extending down toward your left hip.
- Slowly tilt your head to the left, bringing your left ear nearer your left shoulder.
- Hold for 15-30 seconds.
- Gently apply pressure with your right hand to deepen the shoulder stretch.
- Release and return to the starting position.
- Repeat on the opposite side, putting your left hand behind your back and turning your head to the right.
- Perform 2-3 repetitions on each side.

7. Levator Scapulae Stretch:
- Sit or stand with your back straight.
- Reach your right hand over the top of your head and gently move your head toward your right shoulder.
- Hold the stretch for 15-30 seconds.
- Release and repeat on the opposite side, using your left hand to move your head toward your left shoulder.
- Perform 2-3 repetitions on each side.

Remember to practice these stretches slowly and softly, without straining your range of motion. If you encounter pain or discomfort beyond a minor stretch sensation, stop immediately and seek a healthcare expert. Stretching should always be pleasant and never uncomfortable. Incorporating these neck and shoulder exercises into your regular routine will help increase flexibility and alleviate stress in these regions.

- Upper and Lower Back Stretches

Stretching the upper and lower back is vital for maintaining flexibility, decreasing muscular tension, and relieving soreness. Here are helpful upper and lower back stretches to add in your everyday routine:

Upper Back Stretches:

1. Seated Cat-Cow Stretch:
- Sit on a chair with your feet flat on the ground.
- Place your hands on your knees.
- Inhale, arch your back, and push your chest forward (Cow position).
- Exhale, curve your back, and tuck your chin into your chest (Cat position).
- Repeat this moderate rocking motion for 30 seconds to 1 minute.

2. Shoulder Blade Squeeze:
- Sit or stand with your back straight.
- Bring your shoulder blades together, as if you're attempting to squeeze something between them.

- Hold for 10-15 seconds and release.
- Repeat for 2-3 sets.

3. Upper Back Extension:
- Stand with your feet shoulder-width apart.
- Clasp your hands behind your lower back.
- Gently pull your arms and chest upward, pushing your shoulder blades together.
- Hold for 15-30 seconds and release.
- Perform 2-3 repetitions.

Lower Back Stretches:

1. Child's Pose:
- Kneel on the floor with your big toes touching and knees apart.
- Sit back on your heels and stretch your arms forward on the floor.
- Relax your forehead on the ground.
- Hold for 30 seconds to 1 minute, inhaling deeply.

2. Cat-Cow Stretch:
- Start on your hands and knees in a tabletop posture.
- Inhale, arch your back, elevate your head, and gaze ahead (Cow position).
- Exhale, round your back, tuck your chin, and gaze toward your navel (Cat stance).
- Flow between these places for 30 seconds to 1 minute.

3. Knee-to-Chest Stretch:
- Lie on your back with your legs outstretched.

- Bend one knee and pull it toward your chest, gripping it with both hands.
- Hold for 15-30 seconds and move to the other leg.
- Perform 2-3 repetitions on each side.

4. Supine Spinal Twist:
- Lie on your back with your arms spread out to the sides.
- Bend your knees and elevate them off the ground.
- Gently lower both knees to one side while maintaining your shoulders on the ground.
- Hold for 15-30 seconds and switch to the other side.
- Perform 2-3 repetitions on each side.

5. Cat-Cow Stretch in Child's Pose:
- Start in Child's Pose as instructed above.
- Transition to Cat-Cow stretches by sliding your hips backward into your heels and then forward, arching your back and elevating your head.
- Continue this motion for 30 seconds to 1 minute.

Remember to breathe deeply and keep a slow, controlled pace throughout these periods. Do not push your body into unpleasant postures, and stop immediately if you encounter discomfort. Gradually include these upper and lower back exercises into your everyday routine to enhance back health and flexibility. If you have chronic back troubles or significant pain, visit a healthcare expert for help.

- Hip and Leg Stretches

Stretching your hips and legs is vital for developing flexibility, decreasing muscular tension, and maintaining total lower body mobility. Here are helpful hip and leg stretches to add in your everyday routine:

Hip Stretches:

1. Hip Flexor Stretch:
- Kneel on one knee with the other foot in front, forming a 90-degree angle with your front knee.
- Gently move your weight forward to feel a stretch at the front of your hip on the kneeling leg.
- Hold for 15-30 seconds and move to the other leg.
- Perform 2-3 repetitions on each side.

2. Butterfly Stretch:
- Sit on the floor with your feet together, knees bent outward.
- Hold your feet with your hands and gently push your knees toward the floor.
- Hold for 15-30 seconds and release.
- Repeat 2-3 times.

3. Pigeon Pose:
- Begin in a tabletop posture (on your hands and knees).
- Bring one leg forward and position it behind your wrist.
- Extend the other leg behind you.

- Lower your body toward the ground, experiencing a stretch in the hip of the extended leg.
- Hold for 15-30 seconds and move to the other leg.
- Perform 2-3 repetitions on each side.

Leg Stretches:

4. Standing Quad Stretch:
- Stand on one leg.
- Bend your other knee and pull your heel near your buttocks.
- Hold your ankle or foot with your hand.
- Keep your knees close together and maintain proper balance.
- Hold for 15-30 seconds and move to the other leg.
- Perform 2-3 repetitions on each side.

5. Hamstring Stretch:
- Sit on the floor with one leg stretched straight and the other leg bent, with the sole of your foot on your inner thigh.
- Reach forward toward your outstretched leg, maintaining your back straight.
- Hold your foot, ankle, or shin, depending on your flexibility.
- Hold for 15-30 seconds and move to the other leg.
- Perform 2-3 repetitions on each side.

6. Calf Stretch:
- Stand facing a wall or strong object.
- Place your hands on the wall at shoulder height.

- Step one foot back and maintain it straight, pushing your heel into the ground.
- Lean forward, feeling the stretch in your calf.
- Hold for 15-30 seconds and move to the other leg.
- Perform 2-3 repetitions on each side.

7. Seated Leg Extension:
- Sit on the floor with your legs stretched straight in front of you.
- Reach forward toward your toes, keeping your back straight.
- Hold for 15-30 seconds.
- Repeat 2-3 times.

HIP AND LEG COMBINATION STRETCHES:

8. Lunging Hip Flexor Stretch:
- Start in a lunge stance with one foot forward and the other foot stretched straight behind you.
- Gently thrust your hips forward, maintaining your back straight.
- Hold for 15-30 seconds and move to the other leg.
- Perform 2-3 repetitions on each side.

9. Seated Forward Bend with Butterfly Legs:
- Sit on the floor with your legs in a butterfly posture.
- Extend your arms forward, reaching towards your feet.
- Hold for 15-30 seconds.
- Repeat 2-3 times.

10. Runner's Lunge:

- Start in a lunge stance with one foot forward and the other foot stretched straight behind you.
- Lower your upper body toward the ground while maintaining your hands on the ground or on blocks for support.
- Hold for 15-30 seconds and move to the other leg.
- Perform 2-3 repetitions on each side.

As you execute these stretches, try to breathe deeply and keep proper posture. Stretching should be done gently and without pushing your body into unpleasant postures. If you encounter pain, stop immediately and see a healthcare expert. Incorporate these hip and leg exercises into your regular routine to enhance lower body flexibility and minimize muscular strain.

- Arm and Wrist Stretches

Stretching your arms and wrists may help increase flexibility, decrease tension, and avoid pain, particularly if you spend a lot of time using computers or doing repetitive jobs. Here are helpful arm and wrist exercises to add in your everyday routine:

Arm Stretches:

1. Triceps Stretch:
- Stand or sit with your back straight.

- Raise your right arm above and bend your elbow, reaching your hand down your back.
- Use your left hand to gently press on your right elbow.
- Hold for 15-30 seconds and move to the other arm.
- Perform 2-3 reps on each arm.

2. Biceps Stretch:
- Stand or sit with your back straight.
- Extend your right arm forward, palm facing up.
- Use your left hand to gently pull back on your right fingers.
- Hold for 15-30 seconds and move to the other arm.
- Perform 2-3 reps on each arm.

3. Shoulder Stretch:
- Stand or sit with your back straight.
- Extend your right arm over your chest.
- Use your left hand to gently draw your right arm closer to your chest.
- Hold for 15-30 seconds and move to the other arm.
- Perform 2-3 reps on each arm.

Wrist Stretches:

4. Wrist Flexor Stretch:
- Extend your right arm in front of you at shoulder height.
- Bend your wrist so your fingers point toward the floor.
- Use your left hand to gently pull back on your right fingers.
- Hold for 15-30 seconds and move to the other wrist.
- Perform 2-3 repetitions on each wrist.

5. Wrist Extensor Stretch:
- Extend your right arm in front of you at shoulder height.
- Bend your wrist so your fingers point toward the ceiling.
- Use your left hand to gently pull back on your right fingers.
- Hold for 15-30 seconds and move to the other wrist.
- Perform 2-3 repetitions on each wrist.

Combined Arm and Wrist Stretches:

6. Eagle Arms:
- Cross your right arm across your left arm at the elbows, then rotate your forearms so your palms face each other.
- Bring your hands together if feasible, or grip onto your shoulders.
- Lift your elbows slightly, generating a stretch in your upper back and shoulders.
- Hold for 15-30 seconds and swap arm positions.
- Perform 2-3 repetitions on each side.

7. Wrist Circles:
- Extend your arms in front of you.
- Make gentle circles with your wrists in one direction for 15-30 seconds.
- Reverse the direction and create circles for another 15-30 seconds.

8. Finger Stretches:

- Extend your arms in front of you.
- Spread your fingers as wide as possible.
- Hold for 15-30 seconds, then relax.
- Repeat 2-3 times.

As you execute these stretches, concentrate on soft and controlled motions. Never strain your joints or muscles into unpleasant postures. If you suffer discomfort or pain during any stretch, stop immediately. These arm and wrist stretches may be done routinely to increase your range of motion and relieve tension in these regions.

- Full-Body Stretching Sequences

Performing a full-body stretching exercise is a fantastic technique to increase flexibility, alleviate muscular tension, and promote general relaxation. Here's a detailed full-body stretching routine that you may follow:

Warm-Up (5-10 minutes):
Start with a quick warm-up to stimulate blood flow and prepare your muscles for stretching. Light aerobic workouts like brisk walking or jumping jacks might be useful.

Full-Body Stretching Sequence:

1. Neck Stretch (Neck Flexors and Extensors):
- Gently tilt your head to the right, holding for 15-30 seconds.
- Tilt your head to the left and hold for 15-30 seconds.
- Tuck your chin to your chest for 15-30 seconds.
- Look up at the ceiling for 15-30 seconds.

2. Shoulder Roll:
- Roll your shoulders forward in a circular manner for 10-15 seconds.
- Reverse the action and rotate your shoulders backward for 10-15 seconds.

3. Arm Circles:
- Extend your arms out to the sides.
- Make little circles with your arms forward for 15-30 seconds.
- Reverse the direction and form circles backward for 15-30 seconds.

4. Chest Opener:
- Interlace your fingers behind your back.
- Straighten your arms and elevate your chest, pushing your shoulder blades together.
- Hold for 15-30 seconds.

5. Trunk Rotation:
- Sit or stand with your feet shoulder-width apart.
- Twist your torso to the right, stretching your right hand across your body.
- Hold for 15-30 seconds and switch to the other side.

6. Cat-Cow Stretch (Spinal Flexion and Extension):
- Start on your hands and knees in a tabletop posture.
- Inhale, arch your back, and gaze ahead (Cow stance).
- Exhale, round your back, tuck your chin, and gaze toward your navel (Cat stance).
- Flow between these places for 30 seconds to 1 minute.

7. Hamstring Stretch:
- Sit with your legs out in front of you.
- Reach forward toward your toes, keeping your back straight.
- Hold for 15-30 seconds.

8. Quadriceps Stretch:
- Stand on one leg.
- Bend your other knee and pull your heel near your buttocks.
- Hold your ankle or foot with your hand.
- Keep your knees close together.
- Hold for 15-30 seconds and move to the other leg.

9. Calf Stretch:
- Stand facing a wall or strong object.
- Place your hands on the wall at shoulder height.
- Step one foot back and push your heel into the ground.
- Lean forward, feeling the stretch in your calf.
- Hold for 15-30 seconds and move to the other leg.

10. Child's Pose (Lower Back and Hips):

- Kneel on the floor with your big toes touching and knees apart.
- Sit back on your heels and stretch your arms forward on the floor.
- Relax your forehead on the ground.
- Hold for 30 seconds to 1 minute, inhaling deeply.

11. Hip Flexor Stretch (Lunge Position):
- Kneel on one knee with the other foot in front, forming a 90-degree angle with your front knee.
- Gently move your weight forward to feel a stretch at the front of your hip on the kneeling leg.
- Hold for 15-30 seconds and move to the other leg.

12. Butterfly Stretch:
- Sit on the floor with your feet together, knees bent outward.
- Hold your feet with your hands and gently push your knees toward the floor.
- Hold for 15-30 seconds and release.
- Repeat 2-3 times.

13. Pigeon Pose (Hip Stretch):
- Begin in a tabletop posture.
- Bring one leg forward and position it behind your wrist.
- Extend the other leg behind you.
- Lower your body toward the ground, experiencing a stretch in the hip of the extended leg.
- Hold for 15-30 seconds and move to the other leg.

14. Seated Forward Bend:

- Sit on the floor with your legs stretched straight in front of you.
- Reach forward toward your toes, keeping your back straight.
- Hold for 15-30 seconds.

15. Spinal Twist (Lower Back and Hips):
- Sit on the floor with your legs outstretched.
- Bend one knee and cross it over the other leg.
- Twist your body to the side, positioning your opposing elbow outside the bent knee.
- Hold for 15-30 seconds and switch to the other side.

16. Final Relaxation (Savasana):
- Lie on your back with your arms and legs outstretched.
- Close your eyes and take several deep breaths, allowing your body to totally relax.
- Remain in this posture for 2-5 minutes.

Cool Down (5-10 minutes):
End your full-body stretching regimen with a quick cool-down, which might involve moderate walking or mild motions to bring your pulse rate back to normal.

Perform this full-body stretching exercise daily to develop flexibility, decrease muscular tension, and boost relaxation. Remember to breathe deeply and keep proper posture throughout each stretch. If you encounter pain or discomfort, discontinue the stretch immediately and see a healthcare expert if required.

Chapter4: Advanced Stretching Techniques

- Dynamic vs. Static Stretching

Dynamic stretching and static stretching are two separate stretching methods, each with its own purpose and advantages. Understanding the distinctions between them will help you pick the correct sort of stretching for your unique needs:

Dynamic Stretching:

1. Definition: Dynamic stretching includes moving your muscles and joints through a range of motion in a controlled and intentional way. It often comprises

motions that imitate the activity or sport you're practicing for.

2. Purpose: -
Warm-Up: Dynamic stretching is typically utilized as a warm-up before physical exercise. It helps enhance blood flow to the muscles, elevates the heart rate, and prepares the body for more strenuous actions.
   - Improved Mobility: Dynamic stretching may promote joint mobility and flexibility, making it simpler to conduct dynamic motions during sports or exercise.

3. Examples:
   - Leg swings - Arm circles - High knees - Walking lunges
   - Butt kicks - Hip circles
   - Leg crossovers

4. Key Points: - Dynamic stretches should be done in a controlled way, with an emphasis on form and technique.
   - The idea is to progressively expand the range of motion while avoiding severe stretching or bouncing motions.
   - Dynamic stretching is often done for shorter periods (10-15 seconds each repeat) and includes many repetitions.

Static Stretching:

1. Definition: Static stretching includes sustaining a certain stretch posture for a lengthy duration, generally 15-30 seconds or more. It's done without any dynamic motions or bouncing.

2. Purpose: -
Flexibility Improvement: Static stretching is generally used to enhance flexibility by elongating the muscles and connective tissues.
  - Cool-Down: It's typically utilized as part of a cool-down practice after physical exertion to assist relax and stretch muscles.

3. Examples:
  - Touching your toes and holding the stretch
  - Quad stretch - Shoulder stretch - Triceps stretch - Calf stretch - Butterfly stretch

4. Key Points: - Static stretches should be held in a comfortable posture where you feel a moderate tension but no discomfort.
  - Breathe deeply and evenly during static stretches to help relax into the stretch.
  - Avoid bouncing or jerking motions, since they might lead to damage.
  - Static stretching is often done for longer periods (15-30 seconds or more) to enable the muscles to relax and extend.

When to Use Each Type:

- Dynamic Stretching: Use dynamic stretching as part of your warm-up routine before activities that involve agility, speed, or explosive movements, such as sports, jogging, or HIIT exercises. It helps prepare your body for the unique needs of the sport.

- Static Stretching: Use static stretching during your cool-down after physical exercise to help relax and lengthen muscles. You may also integrate static stretching into your normal flexibility regimen to increase total range of motion.

It's crucial to know that current research reveals that static stretching just before strenuous physical exercise may modestly diminish muscular strength and power. Therefore, many experts advocate employing dynamic stretching as a warm-up before athletics and keeping static stretching for post-activity cool-down or independent flexibility exercises.

Ultimately, the decision between dynamic and static stretching relies on your objectives and the environment of your exercise or activity. Combining both methods of stretching may be a well-rounded strategy to increasing flexibility and lower the risk of injury.

- PNF (Proprioceptive Neuromuscular Facilitation) Stretching

Proprioceptive Neuromuscular Facilitation (PNF) stretching is an advanced and extremely effective stretching method used to increase flexibility and range of motion. PNF stretching is a mix of stretching and tightening the targeted muscles. It may be practiced with a partner or on your own, and it's often utilized in rehabilitation and sports training. There are various PNF stretching strategies, with the most prevalent being the "Hold-Relax" method:

The Hold-Relax PNF Stretching Technique:

1. Choose the Muscle to Be Stretched: Identify the precise muscle or muscle group you wish to stretch. PNF stretching is typically utilized for big muscular groups like hamstrings, quadriceps, or hip flexors.

2. Assume the Starting Position: - Position yourself in a comfortable stretching stance that targets the targeted muscle group. For example, if you're targeting your hamstring, lay on your back with one leg extended and the other leg bent.

3. Passive Stretch (10 Seconds): - Begin with a mild passive stretch. Slowly and slowly go into the stretch

position until you feel a moderate tension in the muscle. Hold this stretch for around 10 seconds.

4. Isometric Contraction (6 Seconds): - Next, activate the muscle you're stretching by contracting it isometrically (without altering its length). In the case of the hamstring, aim to force your extended leg into the ground while opposing with your arms or a partner's resistance.

5. Relaxation (30 Seconds): - After the isometric contraction, relax the muscle fully. Allow it to relax and lengthen.

6. Passive Stretch (Increased Range): - Immediately after relaxation, softly and gradually progress deeper into the stretch. You should be able to extend farther than you did originally owing to the muscle's greater flexibility.

7. Hold the Stretch (15-30 Seconds): - Hold this deeper stretch for 15-30 seconds, concentrating on inhaling deeply and relaxing into the stretch.

8. Repeat (2-3 Times):
   - Repeat the whole procedure 2-3 times for the same muscle area, progressively increasing the strain throughout each repetition.

Important Considerations:

- PNF stretching may be strenuous, so it's vital to communicate with your partner if you're practicing partner-assisted PNF stretching, particularly when providing resistance.

- Ensure that you're well warmed up before starting PNF stretching, since it includes deep stretching that might lead to damage if done on cold muscles.

- PNF stretching may be performed for numerous muscle groups and can help increase both flexibility and strength in those areas.

- It's crucial to execute PNF stretching properly to prevent overstretching or straining muscles. If you're new to PNF stretching, try working with a skilled fitness expert or physical therapist to guarantee optimal technique.

- PNF stretching is especially good for athletes, persons recuperating from ailments, and those wishing to increase flexibility dramatically. It's less typically employed in ordinary workout routines because to its intensity and the requirement for a partner in certain circumstances.

- Yoga and Pilates-Based Stretches

Yoga and Pilates are both fantastic disciplines that integrate stretching as a vital component. They provide a broad variety of stretches and exercises to enhance flexibility, balance, strength, and general well-being. Here are some yoga and Pilates-based stretches and exercises:

Yoga-Based Stretches:

1. Downward-Facing Dog (Adho Mukha Svanasana): - A fundamental yoga posture that stretches the whole body, including the hamstrings, calves, shoulders, and back. - Start on your hands and knees, then push your hips forward while straightening your legs and extending your heels toward the ground.

2. Cobra Pose (Bhujangasana): - A backbend that stretches the chest, belly, and spine. - Lie face down, position your hands under your shoulders, and gradually raise your upper body off the ground.

3. Child's position (Balasana): - A peaceful position that stretches the back, hips, and thighs. - Kneel on the floor, lean back on your heels, and extend your arms forward while lowering your forehead to the ground.

4. Seated Forward Bend (Paschimottanasana): - A seated stretch that focuses the hamstrings, lower back, and spine.
   - Sit with your legs out in front of you, hinge at your hips, and reach for your toes while maintaining your back straight.

5. Pigeon Pose (Eka Pada Rajakapotasana): - A hip-opening stretch that also helps with flexibility in the glutes and lower back. - Start in a tabletop posture, pull one knee forward and out to the side, then stretch the opposing leg behind you, then fold forward.

Pilates-Based Stretches:

1. Swan Dive (Pilates Swan): - A Pilates exercise that stretches the whole front of the body. - Lie face down with your arms stretched forward, then raise your head, torso, and arms off the ground while maintaining your legs planted.

2. Spine Stretch (Pilates Spine Stretch Forward): - A sitting Pilates exercise that stretches the spine, hamstrings, and lower back.
   - Sit with your legs outstretched, flex your feet, and reach your arms forward while rounding your back.

3. Single Leg Circle (Pilates Single Leg Circle): - A leg-strengthening and flexibility exercise that also improves hip mobility.

- Lie on your back, elevate one leg toward the sky, and draw circles with your extended leg while maintaining your core engaged.

4. Rolling Like a Ball (Pilates Rolling Like a Ball): - A delightful workout that massages the spine and stretches the back. - Sit in a compact stance, grab your ankles, and roll backward and forth while balancing on your tailbone.

5. Mermaid Stretch (Pilates Mermaid): - A sitting stretch that targets the side of the body and the hip flexors.
   - Sit with one knee bent and the other stretched to the side, then reach your arm above your head and lean to the side.

Both yoga and Pilates provide different positions and routines that may be customized to varied skill levels and fitness objectives. Incorporating these stretches into your normal regimen may enhance flexibility, strength, and general physical well-being. If you're new to yoga or Pilates, consider attending courses or working with a professional teacher to guarantee appropriate form and technique.

- Incorporating Foam Rolling and Mobility Tools

Incorporating foam rolling and other mobility aids into your stretching regimen may be incredibly effective for increasing flexibility, decreasing muscular tension, and promoting general mobility. Here's how you can properly include foam rolling and mobility equipment into your routine:

1. Foam Rolling:

Foam rolling is a self-myofascial release method that helps release muscle knots and enhance tissue suppleness. It's often used before or after stretching or exercise.

Incorporate foam rolling as follows:

- Warm-Up: Begin your workout with a few minutes of mild cardiovascular warm-up, such as jogging or jumping jacks, to stimulate blood flow and prepare your muscles for foam rolling.

- Target Specific Areas: Focus on parts of your body that tend to be tight or strained. Common locations include the calves, quadriceps, hamstrings, glutes, back, and IT bands.

- Roll Slowly: Place the foam roller beneath the desired muscle region and gently roll back and forth over it. Spend additional time on any sensitive or tight regions, which are likely to be trigger points.

- Apply Pressure: Adjust the pressure by changing your body weight. Use your hands and arms to support your body and manage the amount of pressure you exert.

- Breathe Deeply: Maintain calm breathing throughout the foam rolling practice. Deep breaths may assist relax the muscles being rolled.

- Duration: Spend around 1-2 minutes rolling each muscle group. You may do this both before and after your stretching regimen.

2. Mobility Tools (e.g., Lacrosse Balls, Massage Sticks):

In addition to foam rolling, mobility instruments like lacrosse balls or massage sticks may be utilized for more focused muscle release and greater mobility.

Incorporate mobility tools as follows:

- Specific Targeting: Use a lacrosse ball or massage stick to target smaller, harder-to-reach regions, such as the shoulders, neck, and feet.

- Pressure and Rolling: Apply pressure to the desired location and either roll the ball/stick or maintain pressure while making minor movements.

- Breathe and Relax: As with foam rolling, concentrate on calm breathing and allow the tool to relieve tension in the targeted muscles.

- Duration: Spend roughly 1-2 minutes on each location you're targeting with a mobility tool.

3. Integration with Stretching:

Foam rolling and mobility exercises may be added into your stretching regimen for optimal benefit:

- Pre-Stretching: Foam rolling before stretching helps prepare muscles by releasing knots and improving blood flow, making your stretches more effective.

- Intra-Stretching: Use mobility tools between stretches to target particular areas of stress. For example, roll the shoulders with a lacrosse ball before practicing neck and shoulder exercises.

- Post-Stretching: After your stretching practice, you may utilize foam rolling or mobility tools again to remove any leftover tension and encourage relaxation.

4. Frequency:

Consistency is crucial. Aim to integrate foam rolling and mobility tools into your routine consistently, preferably before and after workout sessions or as part of your daily self-care routine.

By integrating foam rolling and mobility tools with your stretching practice, you may increase your flexibility, minimize muscle pain, and boost your general mobility and physical well-being. Remember to utilize good technique and gradually raise the intensity of your self-massage as required. If you're new to these methods, contact a fitness expert or physical therapist to verify you're practicing them appropriately.

Chapter 5: Maximizing the Benefits of Daily Stretching

- Avoiding Common Stretching Mistakes

Avoiding common stretching blunders is vital to ensuring that your stretching exercise is safe, effective, and helpful. Here are some frequent faults to be aware of and how to prevent them:

1. Not Warming Up:
- Mistake: Stretching cold muscles without warming up appropriately might lead to damage.
- Solution: Begin with mild aerobic workouts like running in place or jumping jacks for 5-10 minutes to boost blood flow and raise your body temperature before stretching.

2. Overstretching:
- Mistake: Pushing your muscles and joints too far beyond their normal range of motion may cause injury or muscle strains.
- Solution: Stretch just to the point of moderate tension, not discomfort. Gradually increase the intensity and length of your stretches over time.

3. Bouncing (Ballistic Stretching):
- Mistake: Bouncing during stretches may lead to muscle rips and damage.
- Solution: Use calm, controlled movements throughout your stretches and prevent any bouncing or jerking actions.

4. Holding Your Breath:
- Mistake: Holding your breath may build tension in your muscles and decrease the efficacy of your stretches.
- Solution: Focus on deep, rhythmic breathing. Inhale gently and deeply through your nose as you prepare for the stretch, and exhale slowly through your mouth as you relax into it.

5. Neglecting Muscle Balance:
- Mistake: Focusing on stretching one muscle group while ignoring its opposite muscles might lead to imbalances.
- Solution: Ensure a balanced stretching program that targets all main muscle groups and their antagonists (opposing muscles).

6. Rushing Through Stretches:
- Mistake: Rushing through stretches without holding them for a suitable length of time might decrease their impact.
- Solution: Hold each stretch for at least 15-30 seconds. Consider implementing longer holds for deeper stretches.

7. Incorrect Technique:
- Mistake: Using poor form or technique during stretches may lead to incorrect muscle activation and inadequate stretching.
- Solution: Learn and practice good technique for each stretch. If required, get help from a skilled fitness expert or physical therapist.

8. Ignoring Pain:
- Mistake: Ignoring discomfort while stretching and pushing through it might result in damage.
- Solution: Discontinue any stretch that produces pain, discomfort, or a sharp feeling. Consult a healthcare practitioner if you encounter chronic discomfort when stretching.

9. Skipping Consistency:
- Mistake: Inconsistency in your stretching regimen might restrict its effects.
- Solution: Make stretching a regular part of your daily or exercise regimen. Consistency is crucial for increasing flexibility and avoiding injury.

10. Not Adapting to Individual Needs:
- Mistake: Using a one-size-fits-all strategy to stretch may not meet your individual requirements or restrictions.
- Solution: Customize your stretching program to meet your own objectives, limits, and any specific areas of difficulty.

Remember that stretching should not be unpleasant or uncomfortable. It should feel like a moderate, regulated tension in the muscle being stretched. If you have any medical concerns or injuries, speak with a healthcare practitioner or physical therapist before beginning a new stretching regimen to verify it's safe and suitable for your unique requirements.

- Combining Stretching with Other Forms of Exercise

Combining stretching with other types of exercise is a terrific method to boost your general fitness and flexibility. Here are some pointers on how to properly incorporate stretching into different sorts of workouts:

1. Warm-Up Stretching:
- Before starting any sort of exercise, start with a quick warm-up that involves dynamic stretching. Dynamic stretches like leg swings, arm circles, and hip circles assist boost blood flow, enhance joint mobility, and prepare your muscles for more intensive motions.

2. Yoga and Pilates:
- Yoga and Pilates are fantastic exercises that naturally involve stretching. In these disciplines, stretching is typically a fundamental aspect of the workouts.
- Follow along with yoga or Pilates classes to ensure you're practicing stretches and exercises properly and to receive the full mind-body benefits of these disciplines.

3. Strength Training:
- Incorporate static stretching into your strength training regimen. Stretch the muscles you're working on during your rest periods to avoid muscular stiffness.
- For example, if you're completing a set of squats, complete a quad and hip flexor stretch during your rest time.

4. Cardio Workouts:
- After an aerobic activity, while your muscles are warm, practice static stretches to enhance flexibility and minimize muscular tension.
- Focus on stretches that target the muscle regions you worked throughout your cardio activity.

5. HIIT (High-Intensity Interval Training):
- Include dynamic stretches as part of your HIIT warm-up to prepare your body for intense bursts of exercise.
- After the HIIT training, practice static stretches to enhance flexibility and avoid muscular tightness.

6. Running and Cycling:
- Stretching is especially crucial for runners and cyclists to preserve flexibility and avoid muscular imbalances.
- Incorporate static stretches for the legs, hips, and lower back after your run or bike session. Hold each stretch for at least 15-30 seconds.

7. Swimming:
- Swimming is a fantastic full-body exercise, and stretching may complement it effectively.
- After your swim, complete a series of static stretches that target the shoulders, back, chest, and legs.

8. Cool-Down:
- Regardless of the kind of activity, complete your session with a cool-down that involves static stretching.

Hold each stretch for 15-30 seconds to help relax your muscles and increase flexibility.

9. Flexibility Workouts:
- Dedicate particular workouts or days to concentrate entirely on flexibility and stretching. Yoga and Pilates lessons are fantastic solutions for this purpose.
- You may also construct your own stretching programs targeting regions that require more attention.

10. Listen to Your Body:
- Pay attention to your body's response. If you sense regions of stiffness or muscular discomfort, apply targeted stretching to treat those areas.

Remember that the key to good stretching is consistency. Incorporate stretching into your workout program frequently to increase flexibility, lower the chance of injury, and boost your overall performance. If you're new to stretching or have special objectives, consider visiting a fitness expert or physical therapist to build a personalized stretching strategy.

- Tailoring Your Routine to Specific Goals

Tailoring your stretching regimen to particular objectives helps you to concentrate on the areas that matter most to you. Whether your objectives are connected to flexibility, muscle repair, injury prevention, or boosting sports performance, here's how to design a tailored stretching routine:

1. Identify Your Goals:
- Determine your particular stretching objectives. Are you wanting to increase flexibility, decrease muscular tension, avoid injuries, recuperate from exercises, or boost sports performance?

2. Assess Your Current Flexibility:
- Evaluate your present degree of flexibility and identify areas that need development. You may utilize easy flexibility tests or self-assessment to determine your baseline flexibility.

3. Prioritize Muscle Groups:
- Based on your objectives and evaluation, prioritize the muscle groups or regions that demand the most attention. For example, if you're a runner, you may want to work on leg and hip flexibility.

4. Choose the Right Types of Stretches:
- Select stretching methods that correspond with your aims. For example:
- Static stretching is beneficial for developing general flexibility.
- Dynamic stretching is helpful for warm-ups before sports or activities.

- PNF stretching may be utilized for both flexibility and muscle rehabilitation.
- Yoga or Pilates-based stretches give a comprehensive approach to flexibility and relaxation.

5. Create a Customized Routine:
- Develop a stretching program that involves stretches targeting your primary muscle groups.
- Allocate extra time to stretches for regions that require the greatest work. For example, if you have tight hamstrings, add numerous hamstrings stretches in your regimen.

6. Set a Schedule:
- Decide how frequently you'll conduct your tailored stretching regimen. Consistency is crucial, so aim for at least a couple times a week, if not everyday.

7. Focus on Muscle Imbalances:
- Address muscular imbalances. If one muscle group is much tighter or weaker than its opposite group, integrate particular stretches and exercises to restore the imbalance.

8. Incorporate Recovery Stretches:
- If muscle rehabilitation is a goal, incorporate stretches that help decrease discomfort and increase circulation. These may include moderate stretches, foam rolling, and mobility exercises.

9. Progress Gradually:

- As you work toward your objectives, slowly increase the intensity and length of your stretches. This may require holding stretches for longer durations or deepening your stretches over time.

10. Listen to Your Body:
- Pay careful attention to how your body reacts to your stretching regimen. If you encounter discomfort or pain, alter your program or seek help from a fitness specialist.

11. Track Your Progress:
- Regularly analyze your progress toward your objectives. Have you gained better flexibility, less muscular tension, or enhanced performance?
- Adjust your program as required depending on your success and developing objectives.

12. Seek Professional Guidance:
- If you have particular fitness or sports objectives, try working with a fitness trainer, physical therapist, or yoga teacher. They may give tailored coaching and verify you're employing suitable practices.

Remember that accomplishing your stretching objectives may require time and regular work. Be patient and persistent, and don't push your body too hard to prevent overstretching or injury. A personalized stretching exercise tailored to your unique objectives can help you get the outcomes you seek while increasing general flexibility and well-being.

- Tracking Your Progress and Staying Motivated

Tracking your progress and keeping motivated are crucial components of maintaining a regular and successful stretching regimen. Here are some techniques to help you track your progress and remain motivated:

1. Set Clear and Specific Goals:
- Define your stretching objectives explicitly. Whether it's developing flexibility in a particular muscle region, expanding your range of motion, or lowering muscular tension, having defined objectives offers you something to strive towards.

2. Create a Tracking System:
- Establish a tracking method to document your progress. This might be as easy as maintaining a stretching notebook or utilizing a smartphone app to document your stretching sessions. Note the length, intensity, and how each stretch feels.

3. Take Before and After Photos:
- Periodically take photographs or videos of your stretches. This visual record may help you observe gains in your flexibility and range of motion over time.

4. Use Measurable Metrics:

- Track indicators that are important to your objectives. For example, you may measure how close you are to touching your toes, the number of inches you can reach in a given stretch, or how many degrees you can enhance your joint mobility.

5. Create a Progress Calendar:
- Develop a visible progress calendar or chart. Mark off each day you finish your stretching regimen. Seeing a sequence of steady work may be inspiring.

6. Celebrate Small Wins:
- Celebrate your victories, no matter how minor. Recognizing and praising oneself for attaining milestones may enhance motivation.

7. Vary Your Routine:
- Keep your stretching regimen interesting by incorporating new stretches, methods, or variations. Variety may make your routine more enjoyable and reduce monotony.

8. Set Short-Term and Long-Term Goals:
- Break down your stretching goals into short-term and long-term targets. Short-term objectives assist sustain motivation by giving instant successes, while long-term goals keep you focused on the greater picture.

9. Establish a Routine:
- Make stretching a regular part of your daily or weekly plan. Consistency is crucial to noticing development. Set

definite times for your stretching practices to develop a habit.

10. Find an Accountability Partner:
- Partner with a friend, family member, or exercise companion who shares your objectives or can keep you responsible. You may encourage each other to keep on track.

11. Track Performance Metrics:
- Use performance indicators relevant to your fitness or activity to assess the effect of your stretching program. For example, if you're a runner, monitor gains in your running times or endurance.

12. Seek Professional Guidance:
- Consider working with a fitness trainer, physical therapist, or yoga teacher who can evaluate your development objectively and give professional direction.

13. Stay Informed:
- Continuously educate yourself about stretching methods, the science behind stretching, and the advantages it gives. Learning new knowledge might renew your drive.

14. Visualize Success:
- Spend a few minutes picturing your objectives and thinking how reaching them would positively influence your life. Visualization may boost your dedication and drive.

15. Embrace Plateaus and Setbacks:
- Understand that improvement may not always be linear. There may be plateaus and setbacks along the road. Use these instances as chances to learn and alter your strategy.

16. Reward Yourself:
- Reward yourself as you hit key milestones in your stretching journey. Treat yourself to something you like or engage in a pleasant pastime.

17. Stay Patient and Persistent:
- Remember that development takes time. Stay patient and tenacious in your efforts, and don't get disheartened by slow or occasional failures.

By using these tactics and keeping dedicated to your stretching practice, you may successfully measure your progress and retain the motivation required to attain your flexibility and mobility objectives. Keep in mind that consistency and devotion are the keys to long-term success.

- Tips for Long-Term Success and Maintenance

Maintaining long-term success in your stretching regimen is vital for enjoying the continuous advantages of better flexibility, less muscular tension, and enhanced mobility. Here are some recommendations to help you build a sustainable stretching regimen for the long term:

1. Make It a Habit:
- Consistency is crucial to long-term success. Set a consistent plan for your stretching exercise and make it a non-negotiable element of your daily or weekly routine.

2. Start Slow and Progress Gradually:
- When starting a stretching program, start with moderate durations and intensities. Gradually increase the time and depth of your stretches as your flexibility improves.

3. Listen to Your Body:
- Pay heed to your body's messages. If a stretch seems painful or unpleasant, adjust it or omit it completely. Discomfort is distinct from the slight tension experienced during a stretch.

4. Mix It Up:
- Keep your exercise interesting by integrating a range of stretches and methods. This reduces boredom and enables you to target various muscle areas.

5. Set Realistic Goals:

- Establish attainable stretching objectives that correlate with your current level of flexibility and conditioning. Celebrate modest accomplishments as you advance toward your greater ambitions.

6. Prioritize Recovery:
- Include rest and recuperation days in your routine. Overstretching or excessive reaching may lead to injury. Allow your muscles to rest and adapt to the stretching stimuli.

7. Combine Stretching with Other Activities:
- Integrate stretching into your current exercise program. Pair it with exercises like yoga, Pilates, weight training, or aerobic routines to promote general flexibility and mobility.

8. Create a Relaxing Environment:
- Designate a tranquil and comfortable location for your stretching regimen. Consider playing peaceful music, lighting candles, or utilizing essential fragrances to create a pleasant ambiance.

9. Use Props and Tools:
- Incorporate props like yoga blocks, straps, or foam rollers to improve your stretches and make them more effective. These tools may help you attain deeper stretches.

10. Seek Professional Guidance:

- Consult with a fitness trainer, physical therapist, or yoga teacher to ensure you're practicing appropriate technique and getting tailored coaching.

11. Be Patient:
- Understand that major gains in flexibility and mobility take time. Be patient with yourself and avoid comparing your development to others.

12. Stay Hydrated:
- Adequate hydration is vital for muscular health and flexibility. Drink lots of water before and after your stretching activities.

13. Address Muscle Imbalances:
- Identify and correct any muscular imbalances that may be hurting your flexibility. Include targeted stretches and strengthening exercises to rectify these imbalances.

14. Periodic Assessments:
- Periodically check your flexibility and mobility to measure your development. Reevaluate your objectives and change your routine as required.

15. Share Your Journey:
- Share your stretching adventure with friends, family, or an online community. Sharing your experiences and progress may give encouragement and support.

16. Be Mindful and Present:

- Practice awareness throughout your stretches by concentrating on your breath and the sensations in your body. This may strengthen the mind-body connection and deepen your stretches.

17. Stay Injury-Aware:
- Be mindful of the indicators of overstretching or damage, such as intense pain, prolonged discomfort, or limited range of motion. If you suffer any of these, get medical treatment soon.

18. Adapt as You Age:
- Recognize that your flexibility requirements and capacities may alter with age. Adapt your stretching regimen properly to fit your changing physique.

Long-term success in stretching and maintaining flexibility takes attention, patience, and a balanced approach. By following these recommendations and making stretching a lifetime habit, you may enjoy the advantages of better flexibility and mobility throughout your life.